# About this Book

*Eating Hints* is written for you—someone who is about to get, or is now getting, cancer treatment. Your family, friends, and others close to you may also want to read this book.

You can use this book before, during, and after cancer treatment. It has hints about common types of eating problems, along with ways to manage them.

This book covers:

◆ What you should know about cancer treatment, eating well, and eating problems

◆ How feelings can affect appetite

◆ Hints to manage eating problems

◆ How to eat well after cancer treatment ends

◆ Foods and drinks to help with certain eating problems

◆ Ways to learn more

Talk with your doctor, nurse, or dietitian about any eating problems that might affect you during cancer treatment. He or she may suggest that you read certain sections or follow some of the tips.

> **Rather than read this book from beginning to end,**
> **look at just those sections you need now.**
> **Later, you can always read more.**

# Table of Contents

## Table of Contents *continued*

· · · · · · · · · · · · · · · · · · · · · · · · · · · · · · · · · · · ·

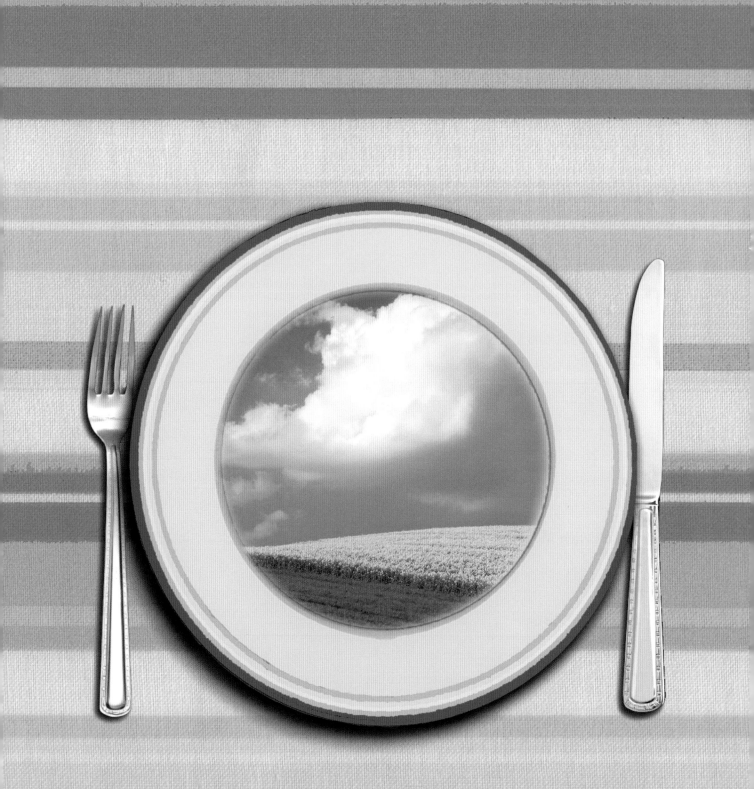

# What You Should Know About Cancer Treatment, Eating Well, and Eating Problems

## People with cancer have different diet needs

People with cancer often need to follow diets that are different from what they think of as healthy. For most people, a healthy diet includes:

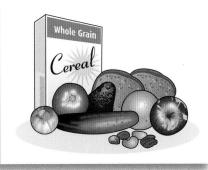

- Lots of fruits and vegetables, and whole grain breads and cereals

- Modest amounts of meat and milk products

- Small amounts of fat, sugar, alcohol, and salt

When you have cancer, though, you need to eat to keep up your strength to deal with the side effects of treatment. When you are healthy, eating enough food is often not a problem. But when you are dealing with cancer and treatment, this can be a real challenge.

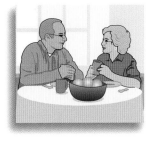

When you have cancer, you may need extra protein and calories. At times, your diet may need to include extra milk, cheese, and eggs. If you have trouble chewing and swallowing, you may need to add sauces and gravies. Sometimes, you may need to eat low-fiber foods instead of those with high fiber. Your dietitian can help you with any diet changes you may need to make.

## Cancer treatment can cause side effects that lead to eating problems

Cancer treatments are designed to kill cancer cells. But these treatments can also damage healthy cells. Damage to healthy cells can cause side effects. Some of these side effects can lead to eating problems. See the list on page 11 to see the types of eating problems that cancer treatment may cause.

Common eating problems during cancer treatment include:

◆ Appetite loss

◆ Changes in sense of taste or smell

◆ Constipation

◆ Diarrhea

◆ Dry mouth

◆ Lactose intolerance

◆ Nausea

◆ Sore mouth

◆ Sore throat and trouble swallowing

◆ Vomiting

◆ Weight gain

◆ Weight loss

Some people have appetite loss or nausea because they are stressed about cancer and treatment. People who react this way almost always feel better once treatment starts and they know what to expect.

## Things to do and think about before you start cancer treatment

◆ Until treatment starts you will not know what, if any, side effects or eating problems you may have. If you do have problems, they may be mild. Many side effects can be controlled. Many problems go away when cancer treatment ends.

◆ Think of your cancer treatment as a time to get well and focus just on yourself.

◆ Eat a healthy diet before treatment starts. This helps you stay strong during treatment and lowers your risk of infection.

◆ Go to the dentist. It is important to have a healthy mouth before you start cancer treatment.

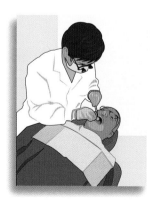

1-800-4-CANCER (1-800-422-6237)

◆ Ask your doctor, nurse, or dietitian about medicine that can help with eating problems.

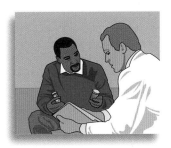

◆ Discuss your fears and worries with your doctor, nurse, or social worker. He or she can discuss ways to manage and cope with these feelings.

◆ Learn about your cancer and its treatment. Many people feel better when they know what to expect. See the list of helpful resources in "Ways to Learn More" starting on page 65.

## Ways you can get ready to eat well

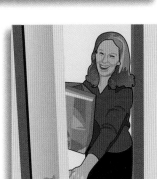

◆ Fill the refrigerator, cupboard, and freezer with healthy foods. Make sure to include items you can eat even when you feel sick.

◆ Stock up on foods that need little or no cooking, such as frozen dinners and ready-to-eat cooked foods.

◆ Cook some foods ahead of time and freeze in meal-sized portions.

◆ Ask friends or family to help you shop and cook during treatment. Maybe a friend can set up a schedule of the tasks that need to be done and the people who will do them.

◆ Talk with your doctor, nurse, or dietitian about what to expect. You can find lists of foods and drinks to help with many types of eating problems on pages 49 to 64.

## Not everyone has eating problems during cancer treatment

There is no way to know if you will have eating problems and, if so, how bad they will be. You may have just a few problems or none at all. In part, this depends on the type of cancer you have, where it is in your body, what kind of treatment you have, how long treatment lasts, and the doses of treatment you receive.

During treatment, there are many helpful medicines and other ways to manage eating problems. Once treatment ends, many eating problems go away. Your doctor, nurse, or dietitian can tell you more about the types of eating problems you might expect and ways to manage them. If you start to have eating problems, tell your doctor or nurse right away.

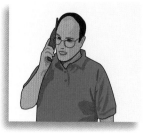

If you start to have eating problems,
tell your doctor or nurse right away.

## Talk with your doctor, nurse, or dietitian about foods to eat

Talk with your doctor or nurse if you are not sure what to eat during cancer treatment. Ask him or her to refer you to a dietitian. A dietitian is the best person to talk with about your diet. He or she can help choose foods and drinks that are best for you during treatment and after.

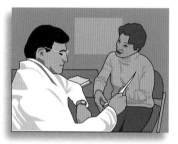

Make a list of questions for your meeting with the dietitian. Ask about your favorite foods and recipes and if you can eat them during cancer treatment. You might want to find out how other patients manage their eating problems. You can also bring this book and ask the dietitian to mark sections that are right for you.

If you are already on a special diet for diabetes, kidney or heart disease, or other health problem, it is even more important to speak with a doctor and dietitian. Your doctor and dietitian can advise you about how to follow your special diet while coping with eating problems caused by cancer treatment.

For more information on how to find a dietitian, contact the American Dietetic Association. See "Ways to Learn More" on page 65 for ways to reach them.

## Ways to get the most from foods and drinks

During treatment, you may have good days and bad days when it comes to food. Here are some ways to manage:

◆ Eat plenty of protein and calories when you can. This helps you keep up your strength and helps rebuild tissues harmed by cancer treatment.

◆ Eat when you have the biggest appetite. For many people, this is in the morning. You might want to eat a bigger meal early in the day and drink liquid meal replacements later on.

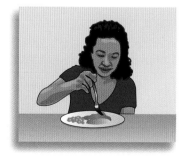

◆ Eat those foods that you can, even if it is only one or two items. Stick with these foods until you are able to eat more. You might also drink liquid meal replacements for extra calories and protein.

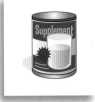

◆ Do not worry if you cannot eat at all some days. Spend this time finding other ways to feel better, and start eating when you can. Tell your doctor if you cannot eat for more than 2 days.

◆ Drink plenty of liquids. It is even more important to get plenty to drink on days when you cannot eat. Drinking a lot helps your body get the liquid it needs. Most adults should drink 8 to 12 cups of liquid a day. You may find this easier to do if you keep a water bottle nearby. Also, try some of the clear liquids listed on page 49.

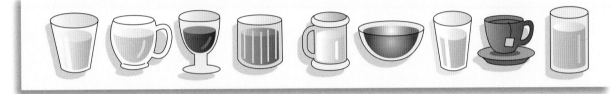

◆ If others are making meals for you, be sure to tell them your needs and concerns.

## Taking special care with food to avoid infections

Some cancer treatments can make you more likely to get infections. When this happens, you need to take special care in the way you handle and prepare food. Here are some ways:

◆ Keep hot foods hot and cold foods cold. Put leftovers in the refrigerator as soon as you are done eating.

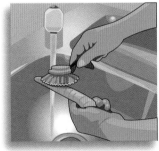

◆ Scrub all raw fruits and vegetables before you eat them. Do not eat foods (like raspberries) that cannot be washed well. You should scrub fruits and vegetable that have rough surfaces, such as melons, before you cut them.

◆ Wash your hands, knives, and counter tops before and after you prepare food. This is most important when preparing raw meat, chicken, turkey, and fish.

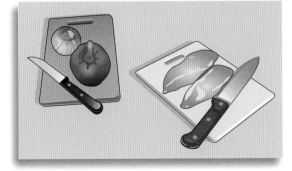

◆ Use one cutting board for meat and one for fruits and vegetables.

- Thaw meat, chicken, turkey, and fish in the refrigerator or defrost them in the microwave. Do not leave them sitting out.

- Cook meat, chicken, turkey, and eggs thoroughly. Meats should not have any pink inside. Eggs should be hard, not runny.

- Do not eat raw fish or shellfish, such as sushi and uncooked oysters.

- Make sure that all of your juices, milk products, and honey are pasteurized.

- Do not use foods or drinks that are past their freshness date.

- Do not buy foods from bulk bins.

- Do not eat at buffets, salad bars, or self-service restaurants.

- Do not eat foods that show signs of mold. This includes moldy cheeses such as bleu cheese and Roquefort.

For more information about infection and cancer treatment, see *Chemotherapy and You: Support for People With Cancer*, a book from the National Cancer Institute. You can get it free by calling 1-800-4-CANCER (1-800-422-6237) or online at www.cancer.gov/publications.

## Using food, vitamins, and other supplements to fight cancer

Many people want to know how they can help their body fight cancer by eating certain foods or taking vitamins or supplements. But, there are no studies that prove that any special diet, food, vitamin, mineral, dietary supplement, herb, or combination of these can slow cancer, cure it, or keep it from coming back. In fact, some of these products can cause other problems by changing how your cancer treatment works.

Talk with your doctor, nurse, or dietitian before going on a special diet or taking any supplements. To avoid problems, be sure to follow their advice.

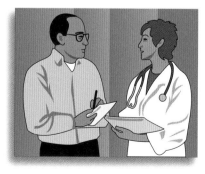

For more information about complementary and alternative therapies, see *Thinking About Complementary & Alternative Medicine: A Guide for People With Cancer*. You can get this book free from the National Cancer Institute. Call 1-800-4-CANCER (1-800-422-6237) or order online at www.cancer.gov/publications.

Talk with your doctor before going on a special diet or taking any supplements. Some vitamins and supplements can change how your cancer treatment works.

## A special note for caregivers

◆ **Do not be surprised or upset if your loved one's tastes change from day to day.** There may be days when he or she does not want a favorite food or says it tastes bad now.

◆ **Keep food within easy reach.** This way, your loved one can have a snack when he or she is ready to eat. You might put a snack-pack of applesauce or pudding (along with a spoon) on the bedside table. Or try keeping a bag of cut-up carrots on the refrigerator shelf.

◆ **Offer gentle support.** This is much more helpful than pushing your loved one to eat. Suggest that he or she drinks plenty of clear and full liquids when he or she has no appetite. For ideas on clear liquids, see page 49, and for full liquids, see page 50.

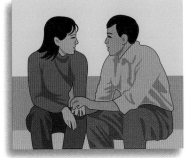

◆ **Talk with your loved one about ways to manage eating problems.** Doing this together can help you both feel more in control.

For more information about being a caregiver, see *When Someone You Love Is Being Treated for Cancer*. You can get this book free from the National Cancer Institute. Call 1-800-4-CANCER (1-800-422-6237) or order online at www.cancer.gov/publications.

# Feelings Can Affect Your Appetite During Cancer Treatment

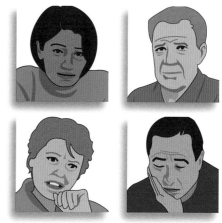

During cancer treatment, you may feel:

◆ Depressed

◆ Anxious

◆ Afraid

◆ Angry

◆ Helpless

◆ Alone

It is normal to have these feelings. Although these are not eating problems themselves, strong feelings like these can affect your interest in food, shopping, and cooking. Fatigue can also make it harder to cope.

## Coping with your feelings during cancer treatment

There are many things you can do to cope with your feelings during treatment so they do not ruin your appetite. Here are some ideas that have worked for other people.

◆ **Eat your favorite foods on days you do <u>not</u> have treatment.** This way, you can enjoy the foods, but they won't remind you of something upsetting.

◆ **Relax, meditate, or pray.** Activities like these help many people feel calm and less stressed.

◆ **Talk with someone you trust about your feelings.** You may want to talk with a close friend, family member, religious or spiritual leader, nurse, social worker, counselor, or psychologist. You may also find it helpful to talk with someone who has gone through cancer treatment.

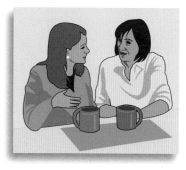

◆ **Join a cancer support group.** This can be a way to meet others dealing with problems like yours. In support group meetings, you can talk about your feelings and listen to other people talk about theirs. You can also learn how others cope with cancer, treatment side effects, and eating problems. Ask your doctor, nurse, or social worker about support group meetings near you. You may also want to know about support groups that meet over the Internet. These can be very helpful if you cannot travel or there is no group that meets close by.

◆ **Learn about eating problems and other side effects before treatment starts.** Many people feel more in control when they know what to expect and how to manage problems that may occur.

◆ **Get enough rest.** Make sure you get at least 7 to 8 hours of sleep each night. During the day, spend time doing quiet activities such as reading or watching a movie.

◆ **Do not push yourself to do too much or more than you can manage.** Look for easier ways to do your daily tasks. Many people feel better when they ask for or accept help from others.

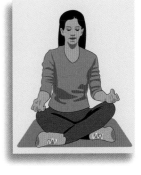

◆ **Be active each day.** Studies show that many people feel better when they take short walks or do light exercise each day. Being active like this can also help improve your appetite.

◆ **Talk with your doctor or nurse about medicine if you find it very hard to cope with your feelings.**

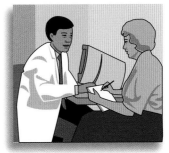

## Ways to learn more

The following groups provide support for people with cancer and their families and friends.

### The Cancer Support Community

Dedicated to providing support, education, and hope to people affected by cancer.

| | |
|---|---|
| Call: | 1-888-793-9355 or 202-659-9709 |
| Visit: | www.cancersupportcommunity.org |
| E-mail: | help@cancersupportcommunity.org |

**CancerCare, Inc.**

Offers free support, information, financial assistance, and practical help to people with cancer and their loved ones.

Call:       1-800-813-HOPE (1-800-813-4673)
Visit:      www.cancercare.org
E-mail:     info@cancercare.org

To read more about ways to cope with your feelings, see *Taking Time: Support for People With Cancer*. To learn more about coping with fatigue caused by cancer treatment, see *Chemotherapy and You* and *Radiation Therapy and You*. These books are from the National Cancer Institute. You can get free copies at www.cancer.gov/publications or 1-800-4-CANCER (1-800-422-6237).

# Eating Problems At-A-Glance

Below is a list of eating problems that cancer treatment may cause. Not everyone gets every eating problem. Some people don't have any problems. Which ones you might have will depend on the type and doses of treatment you receive and whether you have other health problems, such as diabetes or kidney or heart disease.

Talk with your doctor, nurse or dietitian about the eating problems on this list. Ask which ones might affect you. Put a check mark next to the ones you may get or are having now and go to the pages listed to learn more.

| Eating Problems | ✔ Eating problems that you *might* have | Pages to learn more |
|---|---|---|
| Appetite Loss | | 12 |
| Changes in Sense of Taste or Smell | | 15 |
| Constipation | | 17 |
| Diarrhea | | 20 |
| Dry Mouth | | 23 |
| Lactose Intolerance | | 25 |
| Nausea | | 27 |
| Sore Mouth | | 30 |
| Sore Throat and Trouble Swallowing | | 34 |
| Vomiting | | 37 |
| Weight Gain | | 39 |
| Weight Loss | | 41 |

# Appetite Loss

## What it is

Appetite loss is when you do not want to eat or do not feel like eating very much. It is a common problem that occurs with cancer and its treatment. You may have appetite loss for just 1 or 2 days, or throughout your course of treatment.

## Why it happens

No one knows just what causes appetite loss. Reasons may include:

◆ The cancer itself

◆ Fatigue

◆ Pain

◆ Feelings such as stress, fear, depression, and anxiety

◆ Cancer treatment side effects such as nausea, vomiting, or changes in how foods taste or smell

## Ways to manage with food

◆ **When it is hard to eat, drink a liquid or powdered meal replacement (such as "instant breakfast").**

◆ **Eat 5 or 6 small meals each day instead of 3 large meals.** You may find it helps to eat smaller amounts at one time. This can also keep you from feeling too full.

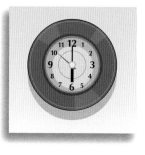

◆ **Keep snacks nearby for when you feel like eating.** Take easy-to-carry snacks such as peanut butter crackers, nuts, granola bars, or dried fruit when you go out. You can find more quick and easy snack ideas on page 57.

◆ **Add extra protein and calories to your diet.** You can find ways to add protein on page 59 and calories on page 63.

◆ **Drink liquids throughout the day—even when you do not want to eat.** Choose liquids that add calories and other nutrients. These include juice, soup, and milk and soy-based drinks with protein. You can find lists of clear liquids on page 49 and full-liquid foods on page 50.

◆ **Eat a bedtime snack.** This will give extra calories but won't affect your appetite for the next meal.

◆ **Change the form of a food.** For instance, you might make a fruit milkshake instead of eating a piece of fruit. There is a recipe on the next page.

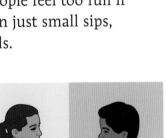

◆ **Eat soft, cool, or frozen foods.** These include yogurt, milkshakes, and popsicles. There is a recipe for banana milkshake on the next page.

◆ **Eat larger meals when you feel well and are rested.** For many people, this is in the morning after a good night's sleep.

◆ **Sip only small amounts of liquids during meals.** Many people feel too full if they eat and drink at the same time. If you want more than just small sips, have a larger drink at least 30 minutes before or after meals.

## Other ways to manage

◆ **Talk with a dietitian.** He or she can discuss ways to get enough calories and protein even when you do not feel like eating.

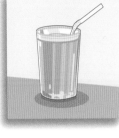

◆ **Try to have relaxed and pleasant meals.** This includes being with people you enjoy as well as having foods that look good to eat.

◆ **Exercise.** Being active can help improve your appetite. Studies show that many people with cancer feel better when they get some exercise each day.

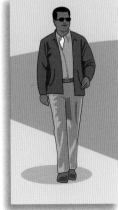

◆ **Talk with your nurse or social worker if fear, depression, or other feelings affect your appetite or interest in food.** He or she can suggest ways to help.

◆ **Tell your doctor if you are having nausea, vomiting, or changes in how foods taste or smell.** Your doctor can help control these problems so that you feel more like eating.

## RECIPE

To help with appetite loss

### Banana Milkshake

1 whole ripe banana, sliced

Vanilla extract (a few drops)

1 cup milk

Put all ingredients into a blender.

Blend at high speed until smooth.

**Yield:** 1 serving

**Serving size:**
Approximately 2 cups

**If made with whole milk:**
**Calories per serving:**
255 calories
**Protein per serving:** 9 grams

**If made with 2% milk:**
**Calories per serving:**
226 calories
**Protein per serving:** 9 grams

**If made with skim milk:**
**Calories per serving:**
190 calories
**Protein per serving:** 9 grams

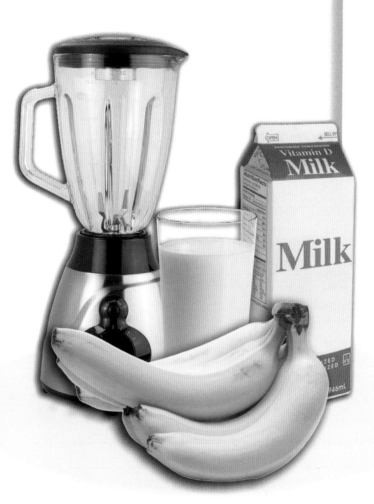

To learn more about dealing with appetite loss, see the section about weight loss on page 41.

# Changes in Sense of Taste or Smell

## What it is

Food may have less taste or certain foods (like meat) may be bitter or taste like metal. Your sense of smell may also change. Sometimes, foods that used to smell good to you no longer do.

## Why it happens

Cancer treatment, dental problems, or the cancer itself can cause changes in your sense of taste or smell. Although there is no way to prevent these problems, they often get much better after treatment ends.

## Ways to manage with food

◆ **Choose foods that look and smell good.** Avoid foods that do not appeal to you. For instance, if red meat (such as beef) tastes or smells strange, then try chicken or turkey.

◆ **Marinate foods.** You can improve the flavor of meat, chicken, or fish by soaking it in a marinade. You can buy marinades in the grocery store or try fruit juices, wine, or salad dressing. While soaking food in a marinade, keep it in the refrigerator until you are ready to cook it.

◆ **Try tart foods and drinks.** These include oranges and lemonade. Tart lemon custard might taste good and add extra protein and calories. But do not eat tart foods if you have a sore mouth or sore throat.

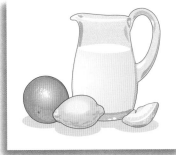

◆ **Make foods sweeter.** If foods have a salty, bitter, or acid taste, adding sugar or sweetener to make them sweeter might help.

◆ **Add extra flavor to your foods.** For instance, you might add bacon bits or onion to vegetables or use herbs like basil, oregano, and rosemary. Use barbecue sauce on meat and chicken.

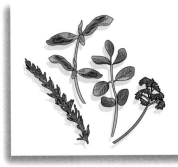

◆ **Avoid foods and drinks with smells that bother you.**
Here are some ways to help reduce food smells:

- Serve foods at room temperature

- Keep foods covered

- Use cups with lids (such as travel mugs)

- Drink through a straw

- Use a kitchen fan when cooking

- Cook outdoors

- When cooking, lift lids away from you

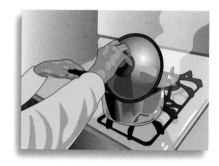

**Eat with plastic forks and spoons if
you have a metal taste in your mouth.**

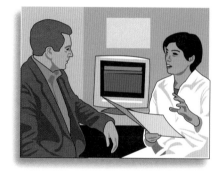

## Other ways to manage

◆ **Talk with a dietitian.** He or she can give you
other ideas about how to manage changes in
taste and smell.

◆ **Eat with plastic forks and spoons.** If you have a metal taste in your mouth,
eating with plastic forks and spoons can help. If you enjoy eating with
chopsticks, those might help, too. Also, try cooking foods in glass pots and
pans instead of metal ones.

◆ **Keep your mouth clean.** Keeping your mouth clean by brushing and flossing
can help food taste better.

◆ **Use special mouthwashes.** Ask your dentist or doctor about mouthwashes
that might help, as well as other ways to care for your mouth.

◆ **Go to the dentist.** He or she can make sure that your changed sense of taste or
smell is not from dental problems.

◆ **Talk with your doctor or nurse.** Tell them about any changes in taste or smell
and how these changes keep you from eating.

# Constipation

## What it is

Constipation occurs when bowel movements become less frequent and stools become hard, dry, and difficult to pass. You may have painful bowel movements, feel bloated, or have nausea. You may belch, pass a lot of gas, and have stomach cramps or pressure in the rectum.

## Why it happens

Chemotherapy, the location of the cancer, pain medication, and other medicines can cause constipation. It can also happen when you do not drink enough liquids or do not eat enough fiber. Some people get constipation when they are not active.

## Ways to manage with food

◆ **Drink plenty of liquids.** Drink at least 8 cups of liquids each day. One cup is equal to 8 ounces. For ideas, see the list of clear liquids on page 49.

◆ **Drink hot liquids.** Many people find that drinking warm or hot liquids (such as coffee, tea, and soup) can help relieve constipation. You might also try

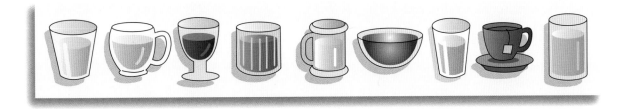

drinking hot liquids right after meals.

◆ **Eat high-fiber foods.** These include whole grain breads and cereals, dried fruits, and cooked dried beans or peas. Try the recipe on page 19. For other ideas, see the list of high-fiber foods on page 55. People with certain types of cancer should not eat a lot of fiber, so check with your doctor before adding fiber to your diet.

Talk with your doctor before taking laxatives, stool softeners, or any medicine to relieve constipation.

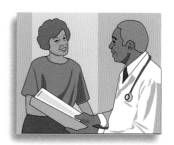

## Other ways to manage

◆ **Talk with a dietitian.** He or she can suggest foods to help relieve constipation.

◆ **Keep a record of your bowel movements.** Show this to your doctor or nurse and talk about what is normal for you. This record can be used to figure out whether you have constipation.

◆ **Be active each day.** Being active can help prevent and relieve constipation. Talk with your doctor about how active you should be and what kind of exercise to do.

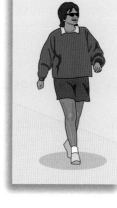

◆ **Let your doctor or nurse know if you have not had a bowel movement in 2 days.** Your doctor may suggest a fiber supplement, laxative, stool softener, or enema. Do not use any of these without first asking your doctor or nurse.

# RECIPE

## To help relieve constipation

## Apple/Prune Sauce

1/3 cup unprocessed bran
1/3 cup applesauce
1/3 cup mashed stewed prunes

**Blend all ingredients and store in a refrigerator.**

Take 1-2 tablespoons of this mixture
before bedtime, then drink 8 ounces of water.

**Note:** Make sure
you drink the water,
or else this recipe
will not work
to relieve constipation.

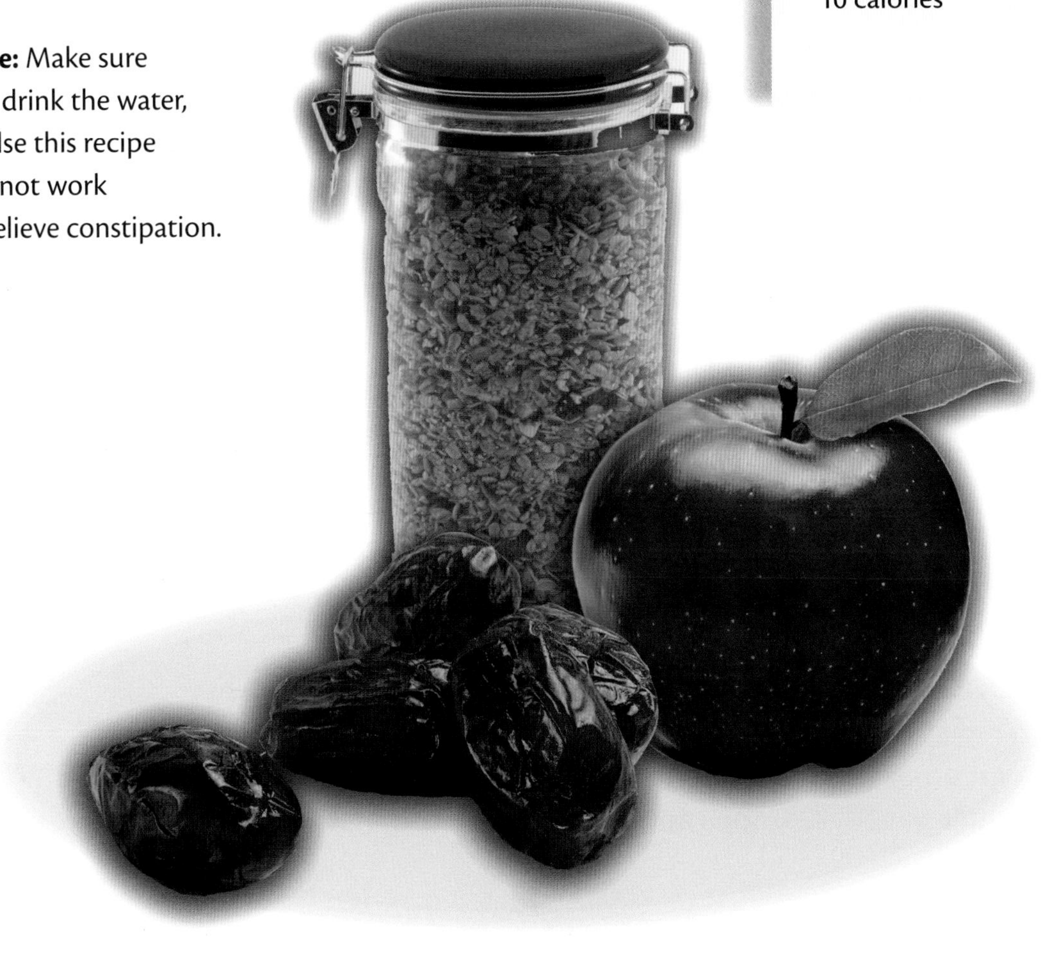

**Yield:**
16 servings

**Serving size:**
1 tablespoon

**Calories per serving:**
10 calories

# Diarrhea

## What it is

Diarrhea occurs when you have frequent bowel movements that may be soft, loose, or watery. Foods and liquids pass through the bowel so quickly that your body cannot absorb enough nutrition, vitamins, minerals, and water from them. This can cause dehydration (which occurs when your body has too little water). Diarrhea can be mild or severe and last a short or long time.

## Why it happens

Diarrhea can be caused by cancer treatments such as radiation therapy to the abdomen or pelvis, chemotherapy, or biological therapy. These treatments cause diarrhea because they can harm healthy cells in the lining of your large and small bowel. Diarrhea can also be caused by infections, medicine used to treat constipation, or antibiotics.

## Ways to manage with food

◆ **Drink plenty of fluids to replace those you lose from diarrhea.** These include water, ginger ale, and sports drinks such as Gatorade® and Propel®. You can see a list of more clear liquids on page 49.

◆ **Let carbonated drinks lose their fizz before you drink them.** Add extra water if drinks make you thirsty or they cause nausea.

◆ **Eat 5 or 6 small meals each day instead of 3 large meals.**

◆ **Eat foods and liquids that are high in sodium and potassium.** When you have diarrhea, your body loses these substances, and it is important to replace them. Liquids with sodium include bouillon or fat-free broth. Foods high in potassium include bananas, canned apricots, and baked, boiled, or mashed potatoes.

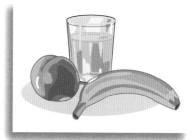

◆ **Eat low-fiber foods.** Foods high in fiber can make diarrhea worse. Low-fiber foods include plain or vanilla yogurt, white toast, and white rice. You can find a list of more low-fiber foods on page 54.

◆ **Have foods and drinks at room temperature, neither too hot nor too cold.**

◆ **Avoid foods or drinks that can make diarrhea worse.** These include:

- Foods high in fiber, such as whole wheat breads and pasta

- Drinks that have a lot of sugar, such as regular soda and fruit punch

- Very hot or very cold drinks

- Greasy, fatty, or fried foods, such as French fries and hamburgers

- Foods and drinks that can cause gas. These include cooked dried beans and raw fruits and vegetables.

- Milk products, unless they are low-lactose or lactose-free

- Beer, wine, and other types of alcohol

- Spicy foods, such as pepper, hot sauce, salsa, and chili

- Foods or drinks with caffeine. These include regular coffee, tea, some sodas, and chocolate.

- Sugar-free products that are sweetened with xylitol or sorbitol. These are found mostly in sugar-free gums and candy. Read product labels to find out if they have these sweeteners in them.

- Apple juice, since it is high in sorbitol

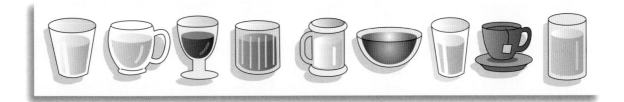

◆ **Drink only clear liquids for 12 to 14 hours after a sudden attack of diarrhea.** This lets your bowels rest and helps replace lost fluids. Let your doctor know if you have sudden diarrhea.

**Ask your doctor or nurse before taking medicine for diarrhea.**

## Other ways to manage

◆ **Talk with a dietitian.** He or she can help you choose foods to prevent dehydration. The dietitian can also tell you which foods are good to eat and which ones to avoid when you have diarrhea.

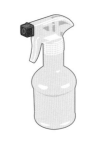

◆ **Be gentle when wiping yourself after a bowel movement.** Instead of toilet paper, clean yourself with wet wipes or squirt water from a spray bottle. Tell your doctor or nurse if your rectal area is sore or bleeds or if you have hemorrhoids.

◆ **Tell your doctor if you have had diarrhea for more than 24 hours.** He or she also needs to know if you have pain and cramping. Your doctor may prescribe medicine to help control these problems. You may also need IV fluids to replace lost water and nutrients. This means you will receive the fluids through a needle inserted into a vein. Do not take medicine for diarrhea without first asking your doctor or nurse.

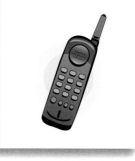

# Dry Mouth

## What it is

Dry mouth occurs when you have less saliva than you used to. This can make it harder to talk, chew, and swallow food. Dry mouth can also change the way food tastes.

## Why it happens

Chemotherapy and radiation therapy to the head or neck area can damage the glands that make saliva. Biological therapy and some medicines can also cause dry mouth.

## Ways to manage with food

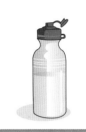

◆ **Sip water throughout the day.** This can help moisten your mouth, which can help you swallow and talk. Many people carry water bottles with them.

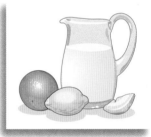

◆ **Have very sweet or tart foods and drinks (such as lemonade).** These help you make more saliva. But do not eat or drink anything sweet or tart if you have a sore mouth or sore throat. It might make these problems worse.

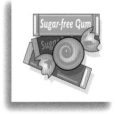

◆ **Chew gum or suck on hard candy, popsicles, and ice chips.** These help make saliva, which moistens your mouth. Choose sugar-free gum or candy since too much sugar can cause cavities in your teeth. If you also have diarrhea, check with your dietitian before using sugar-free products as some sweeteners can make it worse.

◆ **Eat foods that are easy to swallow.** Try pureed cooked foods or soups. You can find a list of foods and drinks that are easy to chew and swallow on page 56.

◆ **Moisten food with sauce, gravy, or salad dressing.** This helps make food easy to swallow.

◆ **Do not drink beer, wine, or any type of alcohol.** These can make your mouth even drier.

◆ **Avoid foods that can hurt your mouth.** This includes foods that are very spicy, sour, salty, hard, or crunchy.

## Other ways to manage

◆ **Talk with a dietitian.** He or she can discuss ways to eat even when a dry mouth makes it hard for you to chew.

◆ **Keep your lips moist with lip balm.**

◆ **Rinse your mouth every 1 to 2 hours.** Mix ¼ teaspoon baking soda and ⅛ teaspoon salt with 1 cup warm water. Rinse with plain water after using this mixture.

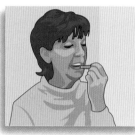

◆ **Do not use mouthwash that has alcohol.** Alcohol makes a dry mouth worse.

◆ **Do not use tobacco products, and avoid second-hand smoke.** Tobacco products and smoke can hurt your mouth and throat.

◆ **Talk with your doctor or dentist.** Ask about artificial saliva or other products to coat, protect, and moisten your mouth and throat. These products can help with severe dry mouth.

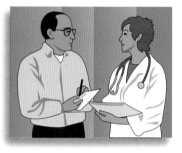

## Ways to learn more

### National Oral Health Information Clearinghouse

A service of the National Institute of Dental and Craniofacial Research that provides oral health information for special care patients. Ask about their booklets, *Chemotherapy and Your Mouth* and *Head and Neck Radiation Treatment and Your Mouth.*

Call:        301-402-7364
Visit:       www.nidcr.nih.gov
E-mail:      nidcrinfo@mail.nih.gov

# Lactose Intolerance

## What it is

Lactose intolerance occurs when your body cannot digest or absorb a milk sugar called lactose. Lactose is in milk products such as cheese, ice cream, and pudding. Symptoms of lactose intolerance can be mild or severe and may include gas, cramps, and diarrhea. These symptoms may last for weeks or even months after treatment ends. Sometimes, lactose intolerance is a life-long problem.

## Why it happens

Lactose intolerance can be caused by radiation therapy to the abdomen or pelvis or other treatments that affect the digestive system, such as surgery or antibiotics.

## Ways to manage with food

◆ **Prepare your own low-lactose or lactose-free foods.** You can find a sample recipe on the next page.

◆ **Choose lactose-free or low-lactose milk products.** Most grocery stores have products (such as milk and ice cream) labeled "lactose-free" or "low-lactose."

◆ **Try products made with soy or rice (such as soy or rice milk and ice cream).** These products do not have any lactose. People with certain types of cancer may not be able to eat soy products. So, ask your dietitian if soy is safe for you to add to your diet.

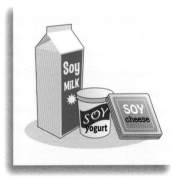

◆ **Choose milk products that are low in lactose.** Hard cheeses (such as cheddar) and yogurt are less likely to cause problems.

## Other ways to manage

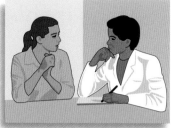

◆ Talk with a dietitian. He or she can help you choose foods that are low in lactose.

◆ Talk with your doctor. He or she may suggest medicine to help with lactose intolerance. These include lactase tablets. Lactase is a substance that breaks down lactose.

## RECIPE

To help with lactose intolerance

### Lactose-Free Double Chocolate Pudding

2 squares baking chocolate (1 ounce each)

1 cup nondairy creamer, rice, soy, or lactose-free milk

1 tablespoon cornstarch

¼ cup granulated sugar

1 teaspoon vanilla extract

Melt chocolate in a small pan.

Measure cornstarch and sugar into a separate saucepan.

Add part of the liquid and stir until cornstarch dissolves.

Add the rest of the liquid.

Cook over medium heat until warm.

Stir in chocolate until mixture is thick and comes to a boil.

Remove from heat.

Blend in vanilla and cool.

**Yield:**
2 servings

**Serving size:**
¾ cup

**Calories per serving:**
382 calories

**Protein per serving:**
1 gram

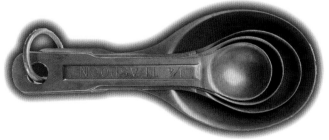

# Nausea

## What it is

Nausea occurs when you feel queasy or sick to your stomach. It may be followed by vomiting (throwing up), but not always. Nausea can keep you from getting the food and nutrients you need. Not everyone gets nausea and those who do may get it right after a treatment or up to 3 days later. Nausea almost always goes away once treatment ends.

## Why it happens

Nausea can be a side effect of surgery, chemotherapy, biological therapy, and radiation therapy to the abdomen, small intestine, colon, or brain. It can also be caused by certain types of cancer or other illnesses.

## Ways to manage with food

◆ **Eat foods that are easy on your stomach.** These include white toast, plain or vanilla yogurt, and clear broth. Try lemon, lime, or other tart-flavored foods. You can see more ideas of foods that are easy on the stomach on pages 52 and 53.

◆ **Eat 5 or 6 small meals each day instead of 3 large meals.** Many people find it easier to eat smaller amounts, more often.

◆ **Do not skip meals and snacks.** Even if you do not feel hungry, you should still eat. For many people, having an empty stomach makes nausea worse.

◆ **Choose foods that appeal to you.** Do not force yourself to eat any food that makes you feel sick.  At the same time, do not eat your favorite foods, so you don't link them to feeling sick.

◆ **Sip only small amounts of liquids during meals.** Many people feel full or bloated if they eat and drink at the same time.

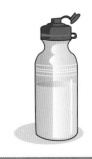

◆ **Have liquids throughout the day.** Drink slowly. Sip liquids through a straw. Or, drink from a water bottle.

◆ **Have foods and drinks that are not too hot and not too cold.** Let hot foods and drinks cool down and cold foods and drinks warm up before you eat or drink them. You can cool hot foods and drinks by adding ice or warm up cold foods in a microwave.

◆ **Eat dry toast or crackers before getting out of bed if you have nausea in the morning.**

◆ **Plan when it is best for you to eat and drink.** Some people feel better when they eat a light meal or snack before treatment. Others feel better when they have treatment on an empty stomach (nothing to eat or drink for 2 to 3 hours before).

**Be sure to tell your doctor or nurse if antinausea medicine does not help.**

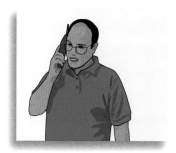

## Other ways to manage

◆ **Talk with your doctor about medicine to prevent nausea** (antiemetics or antinausea medicines). Be sure to tell your doctor or nurse if the medicines are not helping. If one medicine does not work well, your doctor may prescribe another. You may need to take them 1 hour before each treatment and for a few days after. The type of cancer treatment you get and how you react to it affects how long you need to take these medicines. Acupuncture may also help. Talk with your doctor or nurse if you want to try it.

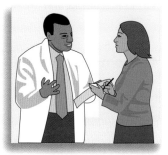

◆ **Talk with a dietitian about ways to get enough to eat even if you have nausea.**

◆ **Relax before each cancer treatment.** You may feel better if you try deep breathing, meditation, or prayer. Many people relax with quiet activities such as reading or listening to music.

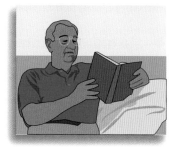

◆ **Rest after meals.** But do so sitting up, not lying down.

◆ **Wear clothes that are comfortable and loose.**

◆ **Keep a record of when you feel nausea and why.** Show this to your nurse, doctor, or dietitian. He or she might suggest ways to change your diet.

◆ **Avoid strong food and drink smells.** These include foods that are being cooked, coffee, fish, onions, and garlic. Ask a friend or family member to cook for you to help avoid cooking smells.

◆ **Open a window or turn on a fan if your living area feels stuffy.** Fresh air can help relieve nausea. Be sure not to eat in rooms that are too warm or stuffy.

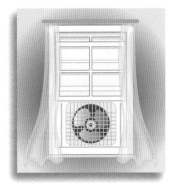

# Sore Mouth

## What it is

Radiation therapy to the head or neck, chemotherapy, and biological therapy can cause mouth sores (little cuts or ulcers in your mouth) and tender gums. Dental problems or mouth infections, such as thrush, can also make your mouth sore.

## Why it happens

Cancer treatments can harm the fast-growing cells in the lining of your mouth and lips. Your mouth and gums will most likely feel better once cancer treatment ends.

## Ways to manage with food

◆ **Choose foods that are easy to chew.** Certain foods can hurt a sore mouth and make it harder to chew and swallow. To help, choose soft foods such as milkshakes, scrambled eggs, and custards. Try the recipe on page 33. For other ideas, see page 56 for a list of foods and drinks that are easy to chew and swallow.

◆ **Cook foods until they are soft and tender.**

◆ **Cut food into small pieces.** You can also puree foods using a blender or food processor.

◆ **Drink with a straw.** This can help push the drinks beyond the painful parts of your mouth.

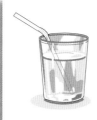

◆ **Use a very small spoon** (such as a baby spoon). This will help you take smaller bites, which may be easier to chew.

◆ **Eat cold or room-temperature food.** Your mouth may hurt more if food is too hot.

◆ **Suck on ice chips.** Ice may help numb and soothe your mouth.

◆ **Avoid certain foods and drinks when your mouth is sore.**
   These include:

   • Citrus fruits and juices, such as oranges, lemons, and lemonade

   • Spicy foods, such as hot sauces, curry dishes, salsa, and chili peppers

   • Tomatoes and ketchup

   • Salty foods

   • Raw vegetables

   • Sharp, crunchy foods, such as granola, crackers, and potato and tortilla chips

   • Drinks that contain alcohol

**If you have a sore mouth, do not use tobacco products or drink alcohol.**

## Other ways to manage

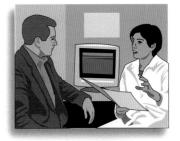

◆ **Talk with a dietitian.** He or she can help you choose foods that are easy on a sore mouth.

◆ **Visit a dentist at least 2 weeks before starting biological therapy, chemotherapy, or radiation therapy to the head or neck.** It is important to have a healthy mouth before starting cancer treatment. Try to get all needed dental work done before your treatment starts. If you can't, ask your doctor or nurse when it will be safe to go to the dentist. Tell your dentist that you have cancer and the type of treatment you are getting.

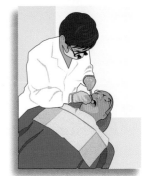

◆ **Rinse your mouth 3 to 4 times a day.** Mix ¼ teaspoon baking soda and ⅛ teaspoon salt with 1 cup warm water. Rinse with plain water after using this mixture.

◆ **Check each day for any sores, white patches, or puffy and red areas in your mouth.** This way, you can see or feel problems as soon as they start. Tell your doctor if you notice these changes.

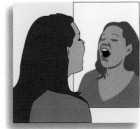

◆ **Do not use items that can hurt or burn your mouth, such as:**

- Mouthwash with alcohol in it

- Toothpicks or other sharp objects

- Cigarettes, cigars, or other tobacco products

- Beer, wine, liquor, or other type of alcohol

◆ **Tell your doctor and dentist if your mouth or gums are sore.** They can figure out whether these are from treatment or dental problems. Ask the dentist about special products to clean and soothe sore teeth and gums.

◆ **Ask your doctor about medicine for pain.** He or she may suggest lozenges or sprays that numb your mouth while eating.

## Ways to learn more

### National Oral Health Information Clearinghouse

A service of the National Institute of Dental and Craniofacial Research that provides oral health information for special care patients. Ask about their booklets, *Chemotherapy and Your Mouth* and *Head and Neck Radiation Treatment and Your Mouth*.

| | |
|---|---|
| Call: | 301-402-7364 |
| Visit: | www.nidcr.nih.gov |
| E-mail: | nidcrinfo@mail.nih.gov |

### Smokefree.gov

Provides resources, including information about tobacco quit lines, a step-by-step smoking cessation guide, and publications to help you or someone you care about quit smoking.

| | |
|---|---|
| Call: | 1-877-44U-QUIT (1-877-448-7848) |
| Visit: | www.smokefree.gov |

## RECIPE

To help with a sore mouth

### Fruit and Cream

1 cup whole milk

1 cup vanilla ice cream or frozen yogurt

1 cup canned fruit (peaches, apricots, pears) in heavy syrup with juice

Almond or vanilla extract to taste

Blend ingredients in a blender and chill well before serving.

**Yield:**
2 servings

**Serving size:**
1½ cups

**If made with ice cream:**

**Calories per serving:**
302 calories

**Protein per serving:**
7 grams

**If made with frozen yogurt:**

**Calories per serving:**
268 calories

**Protein per serving:**
9 grams

# Sore Throat and Trouble Swallowing

## What it is

Chemotherapy and radiation therapy to the head and neck can make the lining of your throat inflamed and sore (esophagitis). It may feel as if you have a lump in your throat or that your chest or throat is burning. You may also have trouble swallowing. These problems may make it hard to eat and cause weight loss.

## Why it happens

Some types of chemotherapy and radiation to the head and neck can harm fast-growing cells, such as those in the lining of your throat. Your risk for a sore throat, trouble swallowing, or other throat problems depends on:

◆ How much radiation you are getting

◆ If you are getting chemotherapy and radiation therapy at the same time

◆ Whether you use tobacco or drink alcohol during your course of cancer treatment

## Ways to manage with food

◆ **Eat 5 or 6 small meals each day instead of 3 large meals.** You may find it easier to eat a smaller amount of food at one time.

◆ **Choose foods that are easy to swallow.** Some foods are hard to chew and swallow. To help, choose soft foods such as milkshakes, scrambled eggs, and cooked cereal.  For other ideas, see page 56 for a list of foods and drinks that are easy to chew and swallow.

◆ **Choose foods and drinks that are high in protein and calories.** See the lists about ways to add protein on page 59 and ways to add calories on page 63. If weight loss is a problem, see the section about weight loss on page 41.

◆ **Cook foods until they are soft and tender.**

- **Cut food into small pieces.** You can also puree foods using a blender or food processor.

- **Moisten and soften foods with gravy, sauces, broth, or yogurt.**

- **Sip drinks through a straw.** This may make them easier to swallow.

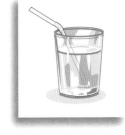

- **Do not eat or drink things that can burn or scrape your throat, such as:**
  - Hot foods and drinks
  - Spicy foods
  - Foods and juices that are high in acid, such as tomatoes, oranges, and lemonade
  - Sharp, crunchy foods, such as potato and tortilla chips
  - Drinks that contain alcohol

**Tell your doctor or nurse if you:**

- **Have trouble swallowing**

- **Feel as if you are choking**

- **Cough while eating or drinking**

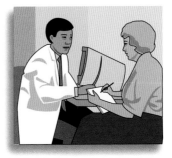

## Other ways to manage

- **Talk with a dietitian.** He or she can help you choose foods that are easy to swallow.

- **Sit upright and bend your head slightly forward when eating or drinking.** Stay sitting or standing upright for at least 30 minutes after eating.

- **Do not use tobacco products.** These include cigarettes, pipes, cigars, and chewing tobacco. All of these can make your throat problems worse.

◆ **Think about tube feedings.** Sometimes, you may not be able to eat enough to stay strong and a feeding tube may be a good option. Your doctor or dietitian will discuss this with you if he or she thinks it will help you.

◆ **Talk with your doctor or nurse.** Tell your doctor or nurse if you have trouble swallowing, feel as if you are choking, cough while eating or drinking, or notice other throat problems. Also mention if you have pain or are losing weight. Your doctor may prescribe medicines to help relieve these symptoms. They include antacids and medicines to coat your throat and control your pain.

## Ways to learn more

### Smokefree.gov

Provides resources, including information about tobacco quit lines, a step-by-step smoking cessation guide, and publications to help you or someone you care about quit smoking.

Call:        1-877-44U-QUIT (1-877-448-7848)
Visit:       www.smokefree.gov

# Vomiting

## What it is

Vomiting is another way to say "throwing up."

## Why it happens

Vomiting may follow nausea and be caused by cancer treatment, food odors, motion, an upset stomach, or bowel gas. Some people vomit when they are in places (such as hospitals) that remind them of cancer. Vomiting, like nausea, can happen right after treatment or 1 or 2 days later. You may also have dry heaves, which occur when your body tries to vomit even though your stomach is empty.

Biological therapy, some types of chemotherapy, and radiation therapy to the abdomen, small intestine, colon, or brain can cause nausea, vomiting, or both. Often, this happens because these treatments harm healthy cells in your digestive track.

## Ways to manage with food

◆ **Do not have anything to eat or drink until your vomiting stops.**

◆ **Once the vomiting stops, drink small amounts of clear liquids (such as water or bouillon).** Be sure to start slowly and take little sips at a time. You can find a list of other clear liquids on page 49.

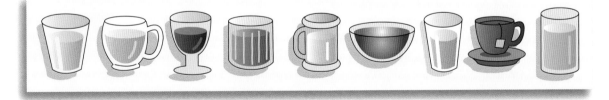

◆ **Once you can drink clear liquids without vomiting, try full-liquid foods and drinks or those that are easy on your stomach.** You can slowly add back solid foods when you start feeling better. There is a list of full-liquid foods on page 50 and a list of foods and drinks that are easy on the stomach on page 52.

◆ **Eat 5 or 6 small meals each day instead of 3 large meals.** Once you start eating, it may be easier to eat smaller amounts at a time. Do not eat your favorite foods at first, so that you do not begin to dislike them.

**Be sure to tell your doctor or nurse if your antinausea medicine is not helping.**

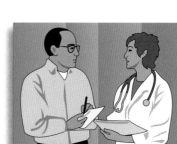

## Other ways to manage

◆ **Talk with a dietitian.** He or she can suggest foods to eat once your vomiting stops.

◆ **Ask your doctor to prescribe medicine to prevent or control vomiting** (antiemetics or antinausea medicines). Be sure to tell your doctor or nurse if the medicine is not helping. Your doctor may prescribe another. You may need to take these medicines 1 hour before each treatment and for a few days after. The type of cancer treatment you get and how you react to it affects how long you need to take these medicines. You may also want to talk with your doctor or nurse about acupuncture. It might also help.

◆ **Prevent nausea.** One way to prevent vomiting is to prevent nausea. You can learn more about nausea on page 27.

◆ **Call your doctor if your vomiting is severe or lasts for more than 1 or 2 days.** Vomiting can lead to dehydration (which occurs when your body does not have enough water). Your doctor needs to know if you cannot keep liquids down.

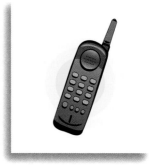

# Weight Gain

## What it is

Weight gain occurs when you have an increase in body weight. Many people with cancer think they will lose weight and are surprised, and sometimes upset, when they gain weight.

## Why it happens

Weight gain can happen for many reasons:

◆ People with certain types of cancer are more likely to gain weight.

◆ Hormone therapy, certain types of chemotherapy, and medicines such as steroids can cause weight gain. These treatments can also cause your body to retain water, which makes you feel puffy and gain weight.

◆ Some treatments can also increase your appetite so you feel hungry and eat more. You gain weight when you eat more calories than your body needs.

◆ Cancer and its treatments can cause fatigue and changes in your schedule that may lead to a decrease in activity. Being less active can cause weight gain.

**Do not go on a diet to lose weight before talking with your doctor about it. He or she will help figure out why you are gaining weight and discuss what you can do about it.**

## Ways to manage with food

◆ **Eat lots of fruits and vegetables.** These are high in fiber and low in calories. They can help you feel full without adding a lot of calories.

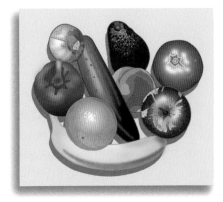

- **Eat foods that are high in fiber, such as whole grain breads, cereals, and pasta.** For more ideas, see the list of high-fiber foods on page 55. People with certain types of cancer should not eat a lot of fiber, so check with your doctor before adding fiber to your diet.

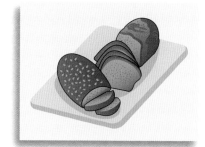

- **Choose lean meats, such as lean beef, pork trimmed of fat, or poultry without skin.**

- **Choose low-fat milk products.** These include low-fat or non-fat yogurt and skim or 1% milk.

- **Eat less fat.** Eat only small amounts of butter, mayonnaise, desserts, fried foods, and other high-calorie foods.

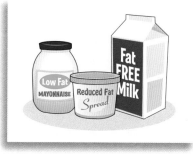

- **Cook with low-fat methods, such as broiling, steaming, grilling, or roasting.**

- **Eat small portion sizes.** When you eat out, take half of your meal home to eat later.

- **Eat less salt.** This helps you not retain water if your weight gain is from fluid retention.

## Other ways to manage

- **Talk with a dietitian.** He or she can discuss ways to limit the amount of salt you eat if your weight gain is from fluid retention. A dietitian can also help you choose healthy foods and make healthy changes to your favorite recipes.

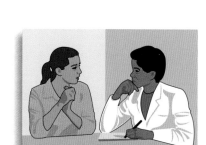

- **Exercise each day.** Not only does exercise help you burn calories, but studies show that it helps people with cancer feel better. Talk with your doctor or nurse about how much exercise to do while having cancer treatment.

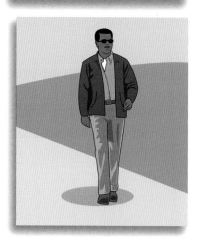

- **Talk with your doctor before going on a diet to lose weight.** He or she can help figure out why you are gaining weight and prescribe medicine (called a diuretic) if you have fluid retention.

# Weight Loss

## What it is

Weight loss is when you have a decrease in body weight.

## Why it happens

Weight loss can be caused by cancer itself, or by side effects of cancer treatment, such as nausea and vomiting. Stress and worry can also cause weight loss. Many people with cancer have weight loss during treatment.

## Ways to manage with food

◆ **Eat when it is time to eat, rather than waiting until you feel hungry.** You still need to eat even if you do not feel hungry while being treated for cancer.

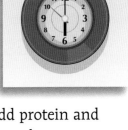

◆ **Eat 5 or 6 small meals each day instead of 3 large meals.** You may find it easier to eat smaller amounts at one time.

◆ **Eat foods that are high in protein and calories.** You can also add protein and calories to other foods. Try the recipe for peanut butter snack spread on page 43. For other ideas, see the lists of how to add protein on page 59 and how to add calories on page 63.

◆ **Drink milkshakes, smoothies, juices, or soups if you do not feel like eating solid foods.** These can provide the protein, vitamins, and calories your body needs. Try the recipe for the high-protein milkshake on page 43. For other ideas, see the list of full-liquid foods on page 50.

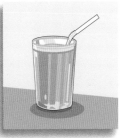

◆ **Cook with protein-fortified milk.** You can use protein-fortified milk (instead of regular milk) when cooking foods such as macaroni and cheese, pudding, cream sauce, mashed potatoes, cocoa, soups, or pancakes. See the recipe for protein-fortified milk on the next page.

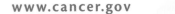

## Other ways to manage

◆ **Talk with a dietitian.** He or she can give you ideas about how to maintain or regain your weight. This includes choosing foods that are high in protein and calories and adapting your favorite recipes.

◆ **Be as active as you can.** You might have more appetite if you take a short walk or do other light exercise. Studies show that many people with cancer feel better when they exercise each day.

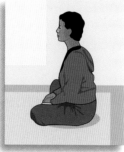

◆ **Think about tube feedings.** Sometimes, you may not be able to eat enough to stay strong and a feeding tube may be a good option. Your doctor or dietitian will discuss this with you if he or she thinks it will help you.

◆ **Tell your doctor if you are having eating problems, such as nausea, vomiting, or changes in how foods taste and smell.** He or she can help control these so you can eat better.

## RECIPES

To help with weight loss

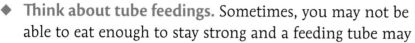
### Protein-Fortified Milk

1 quart (4 cups) whole milk

1 cup nonfat instant dry milk

Pour liquid milk into a deep bowl.

Add dry milk and beat slowly with a mixer until dry milk is dissolved (usually less than five minutes).

Refrigerate and serve cold.

**Note:** If it tastes too strong, start with ½ cup of dry milk powder and slowly work up to 1 cup.

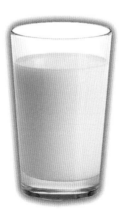

**Yield:** 1 quart

**Serving size:** 1 cup

**Calories per serving:** 211 calories

**Protein per serving:** 14 grams

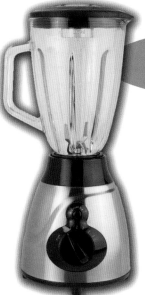

## High-Protein Milkshake

1 cup protein-fortified milk

2 tablespoons butterscotch sauce, chocolate sauce, or your favorite fruit syrup or sauce

½ cup ice cream

½ teaspoon vanilla extract

Put all ingredients in a blender.

Blend at low speed for 10 seconds.

**Yield:** 1 serving

**Serving size:**
Approximately 1½ cups

**Calories per serving:**
425 calories

**Protein per serving:**
17 grams

## Peanut Butter Snack Spread

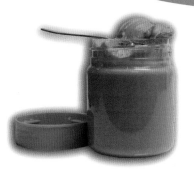

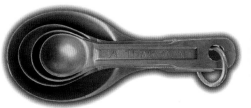

1 tablespoon nonfat instant dry milk

1 tablespoon honey

1 teaspoon water

5 tablespoons smooth peanut butter

1 teaspoon vanilla extract

Combine dry milk, water, and vanilla, and stir to moisten.

Add honey and peanut butter, and stir slowly until blended

Spread on crackers.

Mixture also can be formed into balls, chilled, and eaten as candy.

Keeps well in a refrigerator, but is hard to spread when cold.

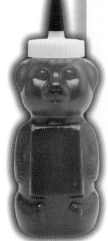

**Yield:** 6 tbsp

**Serving size:** 3 tbsp

**Calories per serving:**
279 calories

**Protein per serving:**
11 grams

# After Cancer Treatment

## Many eating problems go away when treatment ends

Once you finish cancer treatment, many of your eating problems will get better. Some eating problems, such as weight loss and changes in taste or smell, may last longer than your course of treatment. If you had treatment for head and neck cancer or surgery to remove part of your stomach or intestines, then eating problems may always be part of your life.

## Return to healthy eating

While healthy eating by itself cannot keep cancer from coming back, it can help you regain strength, rebuild tissue, and improve how you feel after treatment ends. Here are some ways to eat well after treatment ends:

◆ Prepare simple meals that you like and are easy to make.

◆ Cook 2 or 3 meals at a time. Freeze the extras to eat later on.

◆ Stock up on frozen dinners.

◆ Make cooking easy, such as buying cut-up vegetables from a salad bar.

◆ Eat many different kinds of foods. No single food has all the vitamins and nutrients you need.

◆ Eat lots of fruits and vegetables. This includes eating raw and cooked vegetables, fruits, and fruit juices. These all have vitamins, minerals, and fiber.

◆ Eat whole wheat bread, oats, brown rice, or other whole grains and cereals. These have needed complex carbohydrates, vitamins, minerals, and fiber.

◆ Add beans, peas, and lentils to your diet and eat them often.

◆ Go easy on fat, salt, sugar, alcohol, and smoked or pickled foods.

◆ Choose low-fat milk products.

◆ Eat small portions (about 6 to 7 ounces each day) of lean meat and poultry without skin.

◆ Use low-fat cooking methods, such as broiling, steaming, grilling, and roasting.

## Talk with a dietitian

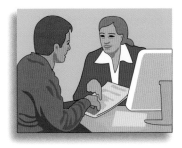

You may find it helpful to talk with a dietitian even when you are finished with cancer treatment. A dietitian can help you return to healthy eating or discuss ways to manage any lasting eating problems.

# Eating Problems That May Be Caused by Certain Cancer Treatments

| Cancer Treatment | What Sometimes Happens: Side Effects |
|---|---|
| **Surgery** | • Surgery may slow digestion (how the body uses food). It can also affect eating if you have surgery of the mouth, stomach, intestines, or throat.<br><br>• After surgery, some people have trouble getting back to normal eating. If this happens, you may need to get nutrients through a feeding tube or IV (through a needle directly into a vein).<br><br>**Note:** Surgery increases your need for good nutrition. If you are weak or underweight, you may need to eat a high-protein, high-calorie diet before surgery. |
| **Radiation Therapy** | Radiation therapy damages healthy cells as well as cancer cells. When you have radiation therapy to the head, neck, chest, or esophagus, you may have eating problems such as:<br><br>• **Changes in your sense of taste** (page 15)<br><br>• **Dry mouth** (page 23)<br><br>• **Sore mouth** (page 30)<br><br>• **Sore throat** (page 34)<br><br>• **Tooth and jaw problems**<br><br>• **Trouble swallowing** (page 34)<br><br>When you have radiation therapy to the abdomen or pelvis, you may have problems with:<br><br>• **Cramps, bloating**<br><br>• **Diarrhea** (page 20)<br><br>• **Nausea** (page 27)<br><br>• **Vomiting** (page 37) |

| Cancer Treatment | What Sometimes Happens: Side Effects |
|---|---|
| **Chemotherapy** | Chemotherapy works by stopping or slowing the growth of cancer cells, which grow and divide quickly. But it can also harm healthy cells that grow and divide quickly, such as those in the lining of your mouth and intestines. Damage to healthy cells can lead to side effects. Some of these side effects can lead to eating problems, such as:<br><br>• **Appetite loss** (page 12)<br><br>• **Changes in your sense of taste** (page 15)<br><br>• **Constipation** (page 17)<br><br>• **Diarrhea** (page 20)<br><br>• **Nausea** (page 27)<br><br>• **Sore mouth** (page 30)<br><br>• **Sore throat** (page 34)<br><br>• **Vomiting** (page 37)<br><br>• **Weight gain** (page 39)<br><br>• **Weight loss** (page 41) |
| **Biological Therapy (Immunotherapy)** | Biological therapy can affect your interest in food or ability to eat. Problems can include:<br><br>• **Changes in your sense of taste** (page 15)<br><br>• **Diarrhea** (page 20)<br><br>• **Dry mouth** (page 23)<br><br><br>*continued on next page* |

| Cancer Treatment | What Sometimes Happens: Side Effects |
|---|---|
| **Biological Therapy (Immunotherapy)** *(continued)* | • **Appetite loss caused by flu-like symptoms, such as muscle aches, fatigue, and fever** (page 12)<br>• **Nausea** (page 27)<br>• **Sore mouth** (page 30)<br>• **Vomiting** (page 37)<br>• **Weight loss, severe** (page 41) |
| **Hormone Therapy** | Hormone therapy can affect your interest in food or ability to eat.<br><br>Problems can include:<br>• **Changes in your sense of taste** (page 15)<br>• **Diarrhea** (page 20) |

# Lists of Foods and Drinks

## Clear Liquids

This list may help if you have appetite loss, constipation, diarrhea, or vomiting.
◆ See page 12 to read more about appetite loss.
◆ See page 17 to read more about constipation.
◆ See page 20 to read more about diarrhea.
◆ See page 37 to read more about vomiting.

| Types | Liquids |
|---|---|
| **Soups** | Bouillon<br>Clear broth<br>Consommé |
| **Drinks** | Clear fruit juices (such as apple, cranberry, or grape)<br>Clear carbonated soda or water<br>Flavored water<br>Fruit-flavored drinks<br>Fruit punch<br>Sports drinks<br>Water<br>Weak tea with no caffeine |
| **Desserts and snacks** | Fruit ices made without fruit pieces or milk<br>Gelatin<br>Hard candy<br>Honey<br>Jelly<br>Popsicles |
| **Meal replacements and supplements** | Clear nutrition supplements (such as Resource® Breeze,)<br>Carnation® Instant Breakfast® juice, and Enlive!®) |

# Full-Liquid Foods

This list may help if you have appetite loss, vomiting, or weight loss.

◆ See page 12 to read more about appetite loss.

◆ See page 37 to read more about vomiting.

◆ See page 41 to read more about weight loss.

| Types | Foods and Drinks |
|---|---|
| **Cereals** | Refined hot cereals (such as Cream of Wheat®, Cream of Rice®, instant oatmeal, and grits) |
| **Soups** | Bouillon<br><br>Broth<br><br>Soup that has been strained or put through a blender |
| **Drinks** | Carbonated drinks<br><br>Coffee<br><br>Fruit drinks<br><br>Fruit punch<br><br>Milk<br><br>Milkshakes<br><br>Smoothies<br><br>Sports drinks<br><br>Tea<br><br>Tomato juice<br><br>Vegetable juice<br><br>Water |

| Types | Foods and Drinks |
|---|---|
| **Desserts and snacks** | Custard (soft or baked) |
| | Frozen yogurt |
| | Fruit purees that are watered down |
| | Gelatin |
| | Honey |
| | Ice cream with no chunks (such as nuts or cookie pieces) |
| | Ice milk |
| | Jelly |
| | Pudding |
| | Sherbet |
| | Sorbet |
| | Syrup |
| | Yogurt (plain or vanilla) |
| **Meal replacement and supplements** | Instant breakfast drinks (such as Carnation® Instant Breakfast®) |
| | Liquid meal replacements (such as Ensure® and Boost®) |
| | Clear nutrition supplements (such as Resource® Breeze, Carnation® Instant Breakfast® juice, and Enlive!®) |

# Foods and Drinks That Are Easy on the Stomach

This list may help if you have nausea or once your vomiting is under control.

◆ See page 27 to read more about nausea.

◆ See page 37 to read more about vomiting.

| Types | Foods and Drinks |
|---|---|
| **Soups** | Clear broth (such as chicken, vegetable, or beef) |
| | All kinds (strain or puree, if needed), except those made with foods that cause gas, such as dried beans and peas, broccoli, or cabbage |
| **Drinks** | Clear carbonated drinks that have lost their fizz |
| | Cranberry or grape juice |
| | Fruit-flavored drinks |
| | Fruit punch |
| | Milk |
| | Sports drinks |
| | Tea |
| | Vegetable juices |
| | Water |
| **Main meals and other food** | Avocado |
| | Beef (tender cuts) |
| | Cheese, hard (mild types, such as American) |
| | Cheese, soft or semi-soft (such as cottage cheese or cream cheese) |
| | Chicken or turkey (broiled or baked without skin) |
| | Eggs |
| | Fish (poached or broiled) |
| | Noodles |
| | Pasta (plain) |
| | Peanut butter, creamy (and other nut butters) |
| | Potatoes, without skins (boiled or baked) |

| Types | Foods and Drinks |
|---|---|
| **Main meals and other food** *(continued)* | Pretzels<br><br>Refined cold cereals (such as corn flakes, Rice Krispies®, Rice Chex®, and Corn Chex®)<br><br>Refined hot cereals (such as Cream of Wheat®)<br><br>Saltine crackers<br><br>Tortillas (white flour)<br><br>Vegetables (tender, well-cooked)<br><br>White bread<br><br>White rice<br><br>White toast |
| **Desserts and snacks** | Angel food cake<br><br>Bananas<br><br>Canned fruit, such as applesauce, peaches, and pears<br><br>Custard<br><br>Frozen yogurt<br><br>Gelatin<br><br>Ice cream<br><br>Ice milk<br><br>Lemon drop candy<br><br>Popsicles<br><br>Pudding<br><br>Sherbet<br><br>Sorbet<br><br>Yogurt (plain or vanilla) |
| **Meal replacements and supplements** | Instant breakfast drinks (such as Carnation® Instant Breakfast®)<br><br>Liquid meal replacements (such as Ensure®)<br><br>Clear nutrition supplements (such as Resource® Breeze, Carnation® Instant Breakfast® juice, and Enlive!®) |

# Low-Fiber Foods

This list may help if you have diarrhea. See page 20 to read more about diarrhea.

| Types | Foods and Drinks |
|---|---|
| **Main meals and other foods** | Chicken or turkey (skinless and baked, broiled, or grilled)<br><br>Cooked refined cereals (such as Cream of Rice®, instant oatmeal, and grits)<br><br>Eggs<br><br>Fish<br><br>Noodles<br><br>Potatoes, without skins (boiled or baked)<br><br>White bread<br><br>White rice |
| **Fruits and vegetables** | Carrots (cooked)<br><br>Canned fruit (such as peaches, pears, and applesauce)<br><br>Fruit juice<br><br>Mushrooms<br><br>String beans (cooked)<br><br>Vegetable juice |
| **Snacks** | Angel food cake<br><br>Animal crackers<br><br>Custard<br><br>Gelatin<br><br>Ginger snaps<br><br>Graham crackers<br><br>Saltine crackers<br><br>Sherbet<br><br>Sorbet<br><br>Vanilla wafers<br><br>Yogurt (plain or vanilla) |

# High-Fiber Foods

This list may help if you have constipation or weight gain.

◆ See page 17 to read more about constipation.

◆ See page 39 to read more about weight gain.

| Type | Foods and Drinks |
|---|---|
| **Main meals and other foods** | Bran muffins<br>Bran or whole-grain cereals<br>Cooked dried or canned peas and beans (such as lentils or pinto, black, red, or kidney beans)<br>Peanut butter (and other nut butters)<br>Soups with vegetables and beans (such as lentil and split pea)<br>Whole-grain cereals (such as oatmeal and shredded wheat)<br>Whole-wheat bread<br>Whole-wheat pasta |
| **Fruits and vegetables** | Apples<br>Berries (such as blueberries, blackberries, and strawberries)<br>Broccoli<br>Brussel sprouts<br>Cabbage<br>Corn<br>Dried fruit (such as apricots, dates, prunes, and raisins)<br>Green leafy vegetables (such as spinach, lettuce, kale, and collard greens)<br>Peas<br>Potatoes with skins<br>Spinach<br>Sweet potatoes<br>Yams |
| **Snacks** | Bran snack bars<br>Granola<br>Nuts<br>Popcorn<br>Seeds (such as pumpkin or sunflower)<br>Trail mix |

# Foods and Drinks That Are Easy To Chew and Swallow

This list may help if you have dry mouth, sore mouth, sore throat, or trouble swallowing.

◆ See page 23 to read more about dry mouth.

◆ See page 30 to read more about sore mouth.

◆ See page 34 to read more about sore throat and trouble swallowing.

| Types | Foods and Drinks |
|---|---|
| **Main meals and other foods** | Baby food<br>Casseroles<br>Chicken salad<br>Cooked refined cereals (such as Cream of Wheat®, Cream of Rice®, instant oatmeal, and grits)<br>Cottage cheese<br>Eggs (soft boiled or scrambled)<br>Egg salad<br>Macaroni and cheese<br>Mashed potatoes<br>Peanut butter, creamy<br>Pureed cooked foods<br>Soups<br>Stews<br>Tuna salad<br>Custard |
| **Desserts and Snacks** | Flan<br>Fruit (pureed or baby food)<br>Gelatin<br>Ice cream<br>Milkshakes<br>Puddings<br>Sherbet<br>Smoothies<br>Soft fruits (such as bananas or applesauce)<br>Sorbet<br>Yogurt (plain or vanilla) |
| **Meal replacements and supplements** | Instant breakfast drinks (such as Carnation® Instant Breakfast®)<br>Liquid meal replacements (such as Ensure®)<br>Clear nutrition supplements (such as Resource® Breeze, Carnation® Instant Breakfast® juice, and Enlive!®) |

# Quick and Easy Snacks

This list may help if you have appetite loss. See page 12 to read more about appetite loss.

| Types of Foods and Drinks | Examples |
| --- | --- |
| **Drinks** | Chocolate milk |
| | Instant breakfast drinks |
| | Juices |
| | Milk |
| | Milkshakes |
| **Main meals and other foods** | Bread |
| | Cereal |
| | Cheese, hard or semisoft |
| | Crackers |
| | Cream soups |
| | Hard-boiled and deviled eggs |
| | Muffins |
| | Nuts |
| | Peanut butter (and other nut butters) |
| | Pita bread and hummus |
| | Pizza |
| | Sandwiches |
| **Fruits and vegetables** | Applesauce |
| | Fresh or canned fruit |
| | Vegetables (raw or cooked) |
| | |
| | *continued on next page* |

| Types of Foods and Drinks | Examples |
|---|---|
| **Desserts and snacks** | Cakes and cookies made with whole grains, fruits, nuts, wheat germ, or granola |
| | Custard |
| | Dips made with cheese, beans, or sour cream |
| | Frozen yogurt |
| | Gelatin |
| | Granola |
| | Granola bars |
| | Ice cream |
| | Nuts |
| | Popcorn |
| | Popsicles |
| | Puddings |
| | Sherbet |
| | Sorbet |
| | Trail mix |
| | Yogurt |

# Ways To Add Protein

This list may help if you have appetite loss, sore throat, trouble swallowing, or weight loss.

◆ See page 12 to read more about appetite loss.

◆ See page 34 to read more about sore throat and trouble swallowing.

◆ See page 41 to read more about weight loss.

| Types | How To Use |
|---|---|
| **Hard or semisoft cheese** | • Melt on:<br>  - Sandwiches<br>  - Bread<br>  - Muffins<br>  - Tortillas<br>  - Hamburgers<br>  - Hot dogs<br>  - Meats and fish<br>  - Vegetables<br>  - Eggs<br>  - Desserts<br>  - Stewed fruit<br>  - Pies<br><br>• Grate and add to:<br>  - Soups<br>  - Sauces<br>  - Casseroles<br>  - Vegetable dishes<br>  - Mashed potatoes<br>  - Rice<br>  - Noodles<br>  - Meatloaf |
| **Cottage cheese/ ricotta cheese** | • Mix with or use to stuff fruits and vegetables<br>• Add to:<br>  - Casseroles<br>  - Spaghetti<br>  - Noodles<br>  - Egg dishes (such as omelets, scrambled eggs, and soufflés)<br><br>*continued on next page* |

| Types | How To Use |
|---|---|
| **Milk** | • Use milk instead of water in drinks and in cooking<br><br>• Use in hot cereal, soups, cocoa, and pudding |
| **Nonfat instant dry milk** | • Add to milk and milk drinks (such as pasteurized eggnog and milkshakes)<br><br>• Use in:<br>  - Casseroles<br>  - Meatloaf<br>  - Breads<br>  - Muffins<br>  - Sauces<br>  - Cream soups<br>  - Mashed potatoes<br>  - Macaroni and cheese<br>  - Pudding<br>  - Custard<br>  - Other milk-based desserts |
| **Meal replacements, supplements, and protein powder** | • Use "instant breakfast powder" in milk drinks and desserts<br><br>• Mix with ice cream, milk, and fruit flavoring for a high-protein milkshake |
| **Ice cream, yogurt, and frozen yogurt** | • Add to:<br>  - Carbonated drinks<br>  - Milk drinks (such as milkshakes)<br>  - Cereal<br>  - Fruit<br>  - Gelatin<br>  - Pies<br><br>• Mix with soft or cooked fruits<br><br>• Make a sandwich of ice cream or frozen yogurt between cake slices, cookies, or graham crackers<br><br>• Mix with breakfast drinks and fruit, such as bananas |

| Types | How To Use |
|-------|-----------|
| **Eggs** | • Add chopped hard-boiled eggs to salads, salad dressings, vegetables, casseroles, and creamed meats<br>• Make a rich custard with eggs, milk, and sugar<br>• Add extra hard-boiled yolks to deviled egg filling and sandwich spread<br>• Beat eggs into mashed potatoes, pureed vegetables, and sauces. (Make sure to keep cooking these dishes after adding the eggs because raw eggs may contain harmful bacteria.)<br>• Add extra eggs or egg whites to:<br>  - Custard<br>  - Puddings<br>  - Quiches<br>  - Scrambled eggs<br>  - Omelets<br>  - Pancake or French toast batter |
| **Nuts, seeds, and wheat germ** | • Add to:<br>  - Casseroles<br>  - Breads<br>  - Muffins<br>  - Pancakes<br>  - Cookies<br>  - Waffles<br><br>• Sprinkle on:<br>  - Fruit<br>  - Cereal<br>  - Ice cream<br>  - Yogurt<br>  - Vegetables<br>  - Salads<br>  - Toast |

*continued on next page*

| Types | How To Use |
|---|---|
| **Nuts, seeds, and wheat germ** *(continued)* | • Use in place of breadcrumbs in recipes<br>• Blend with parsley, spinach, or herbs and cream to make a sauce for noodle, pasta, or vegetable dishes<br>• Roll bananas in chopped nuts |
| **Peanut butter and other nut butters** | • Spread on:<br> - Sandwiches<br> - Toast<br> - Muffins<br> - Crackers<br> - Waffles<br> - Pancakes<br> - Fruit slices<br>• Use as a dip for raw vegetables<br>• Blend with milk and other drinks<br>• Swirl through soft ice cream and yogurt |
| **Meat, poultry, and fish** | • Add chopped, cooked meat or fish to:<br> - Vegetables<br> - Salads<br> - Casseroles<br> - Soups<br> - Sauces<br> - Biscuit dough<br> - Omelets<br> - Soufflés<br> - Quiches<br> - Sandwich fillings<br> - Chicken and turkey stuffings<br>• Wrap in pie crust or biscuit dough as turnovers<br>• Add to stuffed baked potatoes |
| **Beans, legumes, and tofu** | • Add to casseroles, pasta, soup, salad, and grain dishes<br>• Mash cooked beans with cheese and milk |

# Ways To Add Calories

This list may help if you have appetite loss, sore throat, trouble swallowing, or weight loss.

◆ See page 12 to read more about appetite loss.

◆ See page 34 to read more about sore throat and trouble swallowing.

◆ See page 41 to read more about weight loss.

| Types | How To Use |
|---|---|
| **Milk** | • Use whole milk instead of low-fat<br>• Put on hot or cold cereal<br>• Pour on chicken and fish while baking<br>• Mix in hamburgers, meatloaf, and croquettes<br>• Make hot chocolate with milk |
| **Cheese** | • Melt on top of casseroles, potatoes, and vegetables<br>• Add to omelets<br>• Add to sandwiches |
| **Granola** | • Use in cookie, muffin, and bread batters<br>• Sprinkle on:<br>  - Vegetables<br>  - Yogurt<br>  - Ice cream<br>  - Pudding<br>  - Custard<br>  - Fruit<br>• Layer with fruits and bake<br>• Mix with dried fruits and nuts for a snack<br>• Use in pudding recipes instead of bread or rice |
| **Dried fruits (raisins, prunes, apricots, dates, figs)** | • Plump them in warm water, and eat for breakfast, dessert, or snack<br>• Add to:<br>  - Muffins<br>  - Cookies<br>  - Breads<br><br>*continued on next page* |

| Types | How To Use |
|---|---|
| **Dried fruits (raisins, prunes, apricots, dates, figs)** *(continued)* | - Cakes<br>- Rice and grain dishes<br>- Cereals<br>- Puddings<br>- Stuffings<br>- Cooked vegetables (such as carrots, sweet potatoes, yams, and acorn or butternut squash)<br>• Bake in pies and turnovers<br>• Combine with nuts or granola for snacks |
| **Eggs** | • Add chopped hard-boiled eggs to salads, salad dressings, vegetables, casseroles, and creamed meats<br>• Make a rich custard with eggs, milk, and sugar<br>• Add extra hard-boiled yolks to deviled egg filling and sandwich spread<br>• Beat eggs into mashed potatoes, pureed vegetables, and sauces. (Make sure to keep cooking these dishes after adding the eggs because raw eggs may contain harmful bacteria.)<br>• Add extra eggs or egg whites to:<br>  - Custards<br>  - Puddings<br>  - Quiches<br>  - Scrambled eggs<br>  - Omelets<br>  - Pancake or French toast batter |

# Ways To Learn More

**For more resources, see** *National Organizations That Offer Cancer-Related Services* **at www.cancer.gov. In the search box, type in the words "national organizations." Or call 1-800-4-CANCER (1-800-422-6237) for more help.**

## National Cancer Institute (NCI)

Find out more from these free NCI services.

| | |
|---|---|
| Call: | 1-800-4-CANCER (1-800- 422-6237) |
| Visit: | www.cancer.gov |
| Chat: | www.cancer.gov/livehelp |
| E-mail: | cancergovstaff@mail.nih.gov |

## American Dietetic Association

The nation's largest organization of food and nutrition professionals. They can help you find a dietitian in your area.

| | |
|---|---|
| Visit: | www.eatright.org |

## American Institute for Cancer Research

Answers questions about diet, nutrition, and cancer through its "Nutrition Hotline" phone and e-mail service. Has many consumer and health professional brochures, plus health aids about diet and nutrition, and their link to cancer and cancer prevention.

| | |
|---|---|
| Call: | 1-800-843-8114 |
| Visit: | www.aicr.org |
| E-mail: | aicrweb@aicr.org |

## The Cancer Support Community

Dedicated to providing support, education, and hope to people affected by cancer.

Call: 1-888-793-9355 or 202-659-9709

Visit: www.cancersupportcommunity.org

E-mail: help@cancersupportcommunity.org

## CancerCare, Inc.

Offers free support, information, financial assistance, and practical help to people with cancer and their loved ones.

Call: 1-800-813-HOPE (1-800-813-4673)

Visit: www.cancercare.org

E-mail: info@cancercare.org

## National Oral Health Information Clearinghouse

A service of the National Institute of Dental and Craniofacial Research that provides oral health information for special care patients.

Call: 301-402-7364

Visit: www.nidcr.nih.gov

E-mail: nidcrinfo@mail.nih.gov

## Smokefree.gov

Provides resources, including information about tobacco quit lines, a step-by-step smoking cessation guide, and publications to help you or someone you care about quit smoking.

Call: 1-877-44U-QUIT (1-877-448-7848)

Visit: www.smokefree.gov

# Notes

# Notes

1-800-4-CANCER (1-800-422-6237)